Michael Dobe • Boris Zernikow
Editors

Practical Treatment Options for Chronic Pain in Children and Adolescents

An Interdisciplinary Therapy Manual

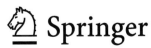

Editors

Michael Dobe
German Paediatric Pain Centre (GPPC)
Children's and Adolescents' Hospital
Witten/Herdecke University
Datteln
Germany

Boris Zernikow
German Paediatric Pain Centre (GPPC)
Children's and Adolescents' Hospital
Witten/Herdecke University
Datteln
Germany

Chair Children's Pain Therapy
and Paediatric Palliative Care
Witten/Herdecke University
School of Medicine
Datteln
Germany

ISBN 978-3-642-37815-7   ISBN 978-3-642-37816-4   (eBook)
DOI 10.1007/978-3-642-37816-4
Springer Heidelberg New York Dordrecht London

Library of Congress Control Number: 2013944046

Printed on acid-free paper

Springer is part of Springer Science+Business Media (www.springer.com)